Can I tell you about Selective Mutism?

Can I tell you about...?

The "Can I tell you about...?" series offers simple introductions to a range of limiting conditions and other issues that affect our lives. Friendly characters invite readers to learn about their experiences, the challenges they face, and how they would like to be helped and supported. These books serve as excellent starting points for family and classroom discussions.

Other subjects covered in the "Can I tell you about...?" series

ADHD

Adoption

Anxiety

Asperger Syndrome

Asthma

Autism

Cerebral Palsy

Dementia

Depression

Diabetes (Type 1)

Dyslexia

Dyspraxia

Eating Disorders

Eczema

Epilepsy

ME/Chronic Fatigue Syndrome

OCD

Parkinson's Disease

Pathological Demand Avoidance Syndrome

Peanut Allergy

Stammering/Stuttering

Stroke

Tourette Syndrome

Can I tell you about Selective Mutism?

A guide for friends, family and professionals

MAGGIE JOHNSON and ALISON WINTGENS
Illustrated by Robyn Gallow

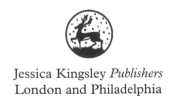

Jessica Kingsley *Publishers*
London and Philadelphia

First published in 2012
by Jessica Kingsley Publishers
73 Collier Street
London N1 9BE, UK
and
400 Market Street, Suite 400
Philadelphia, PA 19106, USA

www.jkp.com

Library of Congress Cataloging in Publication Data
A CIP catalog record for this book is available from the Library of
Congress

British Library Cataloguing in Publication Data
A CIP catalogue record for this book is available from the British
Library

ISBN 978 1 84905 289 4
eISBN 978 0 85700 611 0

Printed and bound in Great Britain by Bell and Bain Ltd, Glasgow

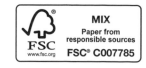

This book is dedicated to all the children and young people with selective mutism with whom we have had the privilege to work. We would like to thank them and their families for all they have taught us. You may even recognise yourselves in this book!

Acknowledgements

Our thanks to Jude Welton for her excellent book
Can I tell you about Asperger Syndrome? which gave
us the inspiration for this book. We are grateful for her
permission to use the format for this sequel on selective
mutism.

We would also like to commend the work of SMIRA*,
and especially Alice Sluckin, OBE, and Lindsay
Whittington, in their tireless support of children, young
people and their families who are living with selective
mutism.

---

* Royalties from this book will be donated to SMIRA (Selective Mutism
Information and Research Association), who provide support and
advice for parents of children with Selective Mutism.

She's Given Up Talking

She's given up talking
Don't say a word
Even in the classroom
Not a dickie bird
Unlike other children
She's seen and never heard
She's given up talking
Don't say a word

You see her in the playground
Standing on her own
Everybody wonders
Why she's all alone
Someone made her angry?
Someone's got her scared?
She's given up talking
Don't say a word

Ah but when she comes home
It's yap-a-yap-yap
Words are running freely
Like the water from a tap
Her brothers and her sisters
Can't get a word in edgeways
But when she's back at school again
She goes into a daze

She's given up talking
She don't say a word
Don't say a word
Don't say a word...

Sir Paul McCartney, 2001

Contents

Introduction 11

Introducing Hannah who has selective mutism 12

Tension, panic and phobia 14

Speaking freely at home 16

It's not refusal to speak 18

Playing with other children 20

Talking in the classroom 22

Feeling stressed and frustrated 24

Speaking with the wider family 26

Associated fears or phobias 28

Telling the class about selective mutism 30

How other children can help 32

What causes selective mutism 36

How teachers can help 37

How parents can help 47

RECOMMENDED READING, DVDs, RESOURCES, WEBSITES
AND ORGANISATIONS 53

Introduction

This book has been written to help everyone understand selective mutism (SM) better:

- Children and young people can read about the difficulties faced by a child with SM. It tells them what SM is, what it feels like to have SM, and how they can help.

- It is a useful, friendly book to share with children with SM to help them understand and talk about how it affects them. It may also help older children with SM talk about their past and present experiences.

- And, of course, adults can learn a lot about SM too!

Extra sections at the back give tips for how teachers and parents can help children with SM. Not all ideas will be necessary for every child; they can be adapted to suit individuals and, of course, many of them will already be familiar.

Readers may wonder why Hannah has SM. There is no single cause. But as with other phobias there will be a combination of an already anxious child and an unfortunate situation, and then the expectation to talk.

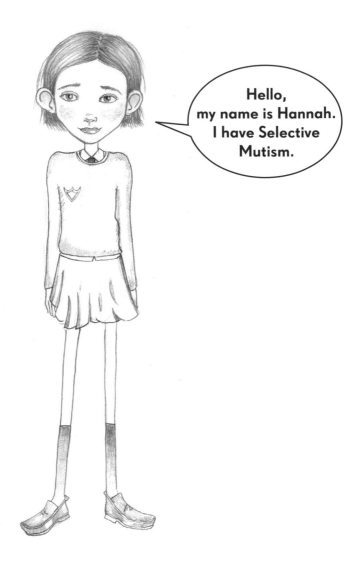

"Some people call it SM for short.
I'd like to tell you what it is, what
it feels like, and how you might
help me – if you want to."

"You can't see that I have selective mutism. I look like most other girls. But you might notice things about me that are a bit different. This is because SM can sometimes make me behave and talk in a way that you might not expect. Like everyone else, people with SM are individuals, and SM affects each person a bit differently. So other children with SM will be like me in lots of ways, but not exactly the same.

The main thing about SM is that I can't talk comfortably with people in every situation. If I'm at home with my parents and close family, I'm fine, and you wouldn't think I had any problem. But if we go out and other people are around – or people I don't know well come to my home – I get anxious and the words can't come out. It's worst when I am at school, because it's full of people I don't know well."

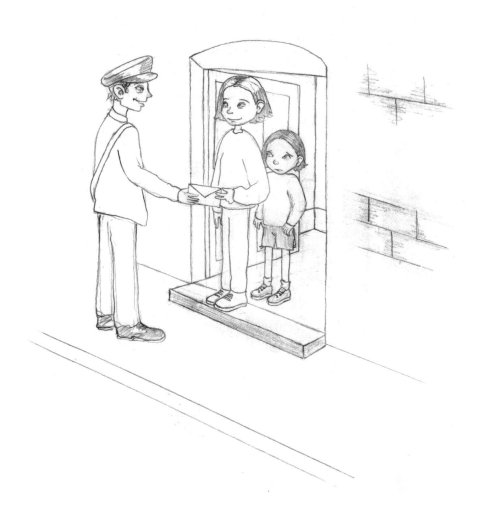

"When someone speaks to me
I get very tense and panicky."

"You may have noticed that when people talk to me I sometimes look rather stiff and my face or my whole body seems frozen. My mum says I look like a rabbit trapped in the headlights. It's true – I feel stuck and can't move. My heart beats fast, I can't breathe easily and my throat goes tight. I can't even turn my head from side to side comfortably. They say adults can get 'panic attacks' and that's just what it feels like.

You know some people can't bear to fly in a plane, or they are petrified of spiders. Well, it's a bit the same with me when I need to speak out. I have a sort of phobia about talking. I feel like there's a spotlight on me.

So I try and avoid times when I might have to speak. It's such a relief to stop trying and not feel anxious. The trouble is, the more I avoid talking the harder it seems to get to start talking."

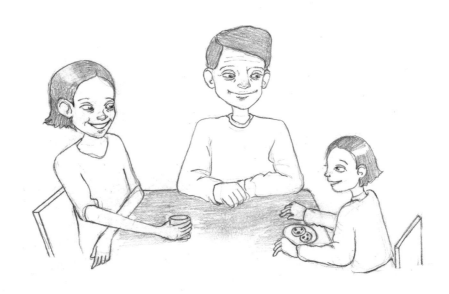

"Because I'm silent you may think
I can't speak at all, or don't speak
English, or that I'm just shy."

"As I said, I can speak fine at home – in fact, I can speak to my mum and dad anywhere if I'm sure no one else will hear us. You can ask them. If I couldn't speak at all, or just didn't know English, it wouldn't be called SM.

In other situations – when I'm in new places or with new people – I can nod or shake my head a bit if someone asks me a question, which proves I understand OK. And sometimes I point too. I have what I'd like to say in my head, and sometimes I know the answer in class before anyone else; but I just can't speak out.

It's a bit like severe shyness but not the same. If I know I'm not expected to speak, I feel fine and I can join in. My panics happen when I have to speak. And it makes it worse if people keep on trying to get me to talk, however nicely they try to do it."

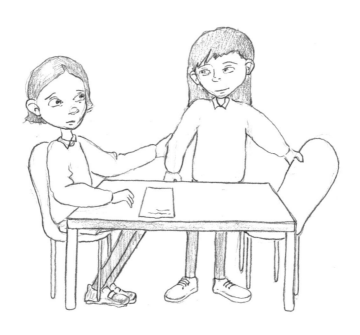

"It upsets me when people
say I am refusing to talk or
trying to get my own way."

"Sometimes grown-ups, and children, think that I do it on purpose – that I am choosing not to talk. I think they think I want to be difficult or get back at them or something. It's not at all like that. I'd love to speak. I just can't get over this fear of talking, and I can't get started.

To make it easier at school, I try to find out exactly what's going to happen and get my friend Maya to sit with me. At first my teacher thought I was trying to take over – but now he realises that it makes me less anxious.

Of course, I might not answer my mum sometimes if I am cross with her or I've done something wrong – don't we all do that?! But that feels completely different to when I can't speak out because of my SM."

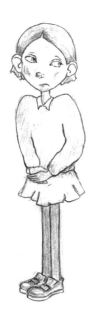
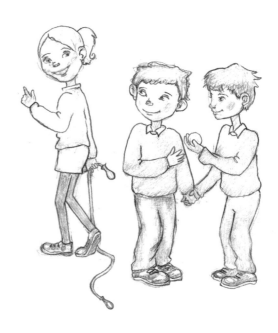

"I'd like to play or join in things more,
but I can't if it means I have to talk."

"In the playground I used to feel very sad and left out. I stood on the edge and watched everyone else having fun. Now I am getting a bit more relaxed. It helps when the other children ask me to join in with their games. I can do the ones where you don't have to talk. Or I go into the corner under the trees with my friend Maya and she talks to me a bit.

I get really worried when I'm asked to a party. I'd love to go but I'm afraid the friend's mum and any new children won't understand my SM.

Maya came to my flat and I liked showing her my room. We played and had a drink. I think Maya was really surprised to hear me talking to my mum! My mum said perhaps I can start going round to her place to play. That made me feel scared so Mum said she'd come with me at first."

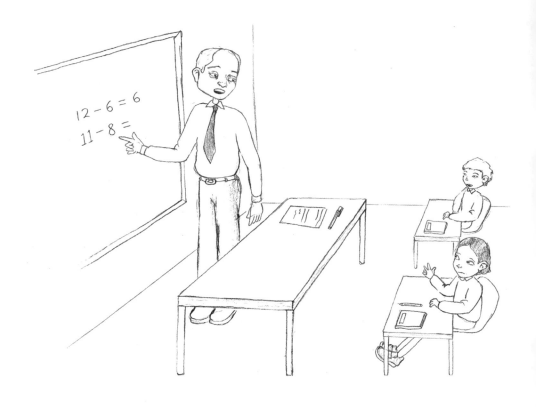

"Talking in the classroom
is very hard for me."

"In class it's OK if we don't have to speak or I can do something that the other children plan. I'm good at maths and sometimes I can join in by using my fingers to give the answer. Or I can join in drawing or painting projects, and I'm starting to write more.

I used to dread it when the teacher said 'Find a partner' or 'Get into groups' – I thought I'd be left out and I never knew what I'd be asked to do or who I'd be with. I don't blame the children for not wanting to be with me, but I felt really sad inside.

Last week my teacher, Mr Bailey, explained to me that I don't have to talk till I'm ready. He said that until then there are other ways I can join in and I can show what I've learned in my writing or my drawing. That's such a relief – it gave me a really good feeling."

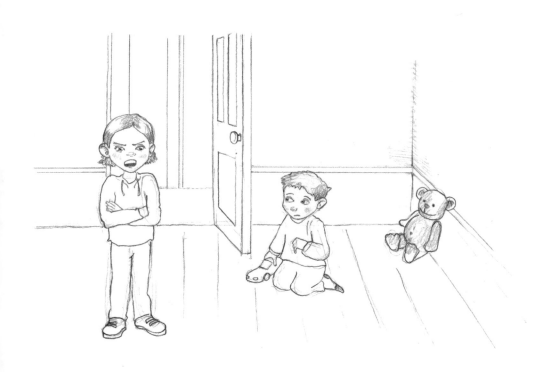

"Sometimes I feel really
stressed and frustrated
because I can't speak out."

"When I'm at school, I feel I always have to be on the lookout for whether I might be expected to talk. And at the same time I have lots of thoughts, ideas, questions and answers that I can't get out. I also try to be brave and not show my feelings. All this makes me very tired by the end of the day.

When I get home, I'm full of all these feelings that I've been bottling up. Then it's like the top comes off the bottle and I can get really cross. It's like I haven't been able to control anything at school – so I have to make up for it by being in charge at home. My mum and my little brother get the worst of it.

On some days it's not so bad and I just do lots of talking when I get home. I suppose I might be a bit bossy, but I don't get into a temper."

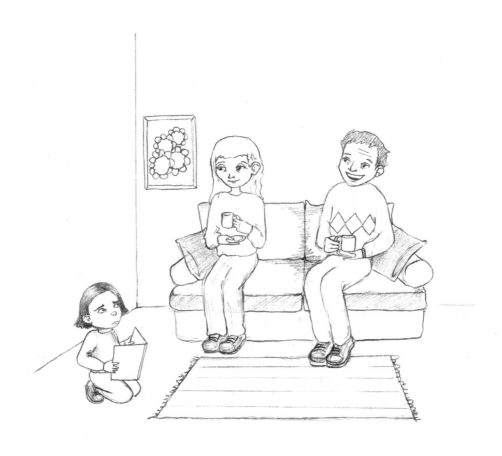

"I wish I could speak comfortably
with my uncle and auntie."

"As well as my mum and dad, my little brother and my big sister, I can talk to Grandma in her home and mine. I see a lot of her and she used to look after me when I was little and my mum was working.

But with others in the family it's not so easy. I find it hard to talk to Gran and Granddad and I know Dad would like me to speak more to them.

I have one uncle who I don't see much. And when I do, he's always asking, 'Why don't you talk to me?' which makes me feel worse. He and my auntie are nice and funny so I wish I could. In the summer they had a baby who can now sit up. Last time they all came round I went and played with the baby – I could talk to him when no one was looking. Perhaps this ll be a start to me talking more with my uncle and auntie."

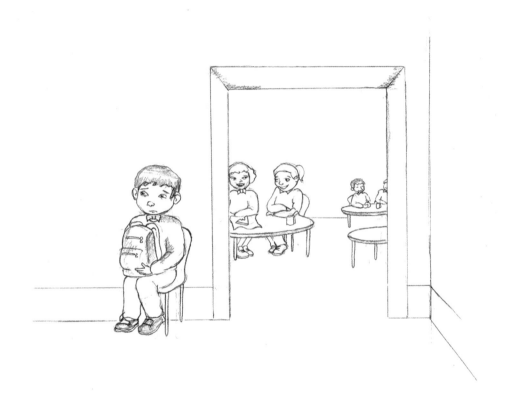

"My mum told me that some children with SM have other fears or phobias."

"I heard that there's a boy in Nursery who has SM too. He's got the same sort of difficulty as me with talking out comfortably. But my mum says he's got other problems – he can't go the toilet or eat his dinner in school. His mum takes him home in the middle of the day to do these things. It's lucky they live round the back of our school!

It must be awful not being able to do these things too. But I suppose it's a bit like our talking difficulty, and not liking people watching or listening to you.

I hope they can help him. I'm sure as he gets older he'll be able to do it bit by bit.

That's how I'm starting to talk – last week I said a few words very quietly to Miss King, our classroom assistant.

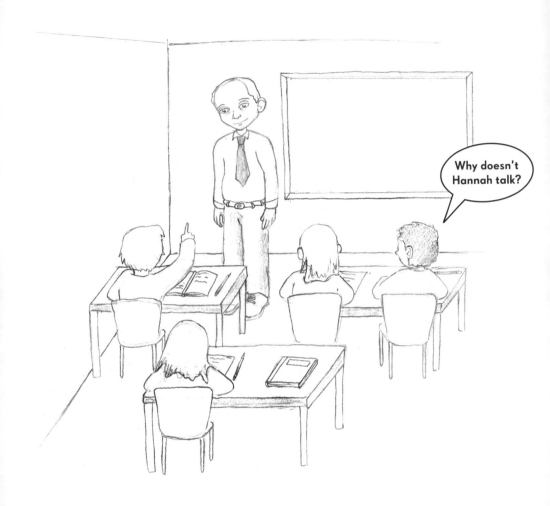

"My teacher tried to answer the other children's questions about SM. I wanted to be there too."

"When we were sharing about how we felt about being in our new class and what made us scared, Mr Bailey told the children that SM is caused by anxiety. He said it's always been difficult for me to talk comfortably with new people in new places, so coming to school was very hard. He explained that there are lots of children with SM, but more girls than boys.

I liked it when he told them I'm starting to get over it and said, 'We're going to help Hannah.' He said that if they don't pester me to talk, I can stop worrying and have fun at school. He talked about small steps so little by little I'll be able to talk to more people.

I felt much better once he'd said all this. Mr Bailey's chosen me, Maya and a new boy to tidy up the classroom every Wednesday playtime, which I'm really pleased about."

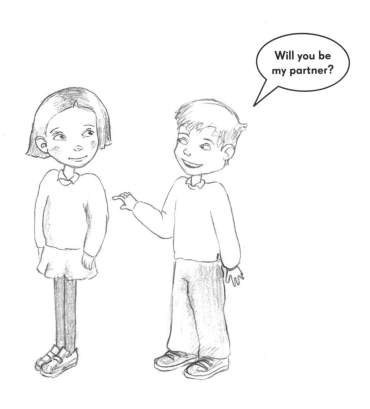

"My mum and I wrote down how my classmates could help me, and Mr Bailey read it out to them."

"Please try and treat me like anyone else and don't make a big thing of my SM.

- Understand that I'm not being rude or unfriendly if I don't talk.

- Please talk to me even though I might not be able to talk back.

- I like it when you save me a place and ask me to sit with you.

- Please invite me to join in or be your partner.

- Please don't ask me too many questions. I like it when you show me things or tell me your news.

- Don't comment or act surprised if I start to talk...

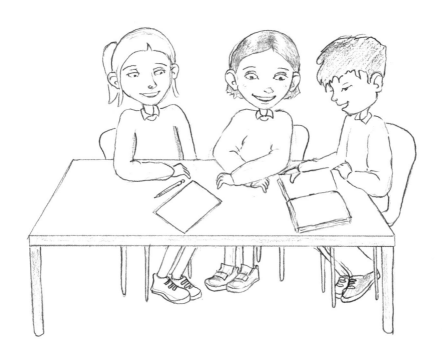

"I feel much happier now
everyone understands."

- Don't laugh or tease me about my difficulty talking – I feel bad enough about it already.

- I'd like to do more by myself – it helps if you do things *with* me, but please don't do them *for* me!

- When I'm practising my small steps targets, I may need to ask you to join in.

- Perhaps you could come to the swings with me and my mum after school.

- I like school, and with your help I think I'll like it even more! I am looking forward to when I can speak comfortably with you all."

What causes Selective Mutism

"You may wonder why I've got SM. I asked my Mum this question and she said there is no one cause – it's a bit different for each child. She said I always hung back and was afraid to try new things. And it was especially hard for me starting playgroup. I panicked when Mum left me on my own and I couldn't talk to the lady who tried to help me to join in. I was never quite the same with new people after that.

My Mum sometimes tells other people that SM is a sort of phobia, which is a word for being REALLY scared of something even though there's no need to be. Some children panic when they see dogs or clowns; and some grown-ups can't fly in a plane. So SM is a phobia of talking to certain people.

Mum says SM starts like other phobias start, and something happens which makes you link horrid panicky feelings to a 'trigger'. With SM the trigger is having to talk to certain people. Children with SM are sensitive and have usually been worriers since they were little, so quite ordinary things can make them panic – being in an unfamilliar place, getting told off, being startled by a stranger. If there's a focus on talking at the same time, talking can become the thing to be scared of."

How teachers can help

(useful for parents too!)

IMPORTANT THINGS TO REMEMBER

"Please try and be as understanding and caring as you can, and remember:

- I can't talk because I've got a sort of talking phobia. I just freeze when I know certain people are listening to me.

- It's not that I'm refusing to talk or I don't want to. I'd love to speak out comfortably.

- As far as you can, please treat me like everyone else and don't draw attention to me.

- Try not to be worried yourself because I can't talk yet – it's not your fault.

- And don't feel you have to get me to speak – I can feel that pressure and it makes it worse.

- I'd really like to know you like me as I am and can see that there are some other things I can do well.

- My mum says I won't always have this difficulty and that little by little I'll take steps to talk out more."

TALKING AND LISTENING

"The way you speak to me makes a difference to how easy it is for me to listen and to talk.

- Please let me know you understand and that when you say hello or chat to me, you don't expect me to talk back. If there's no pressure for me to talk, it's more likely that the words might come out.

- I feel comfortable when you are chatty – talk to me in a normal way, show and tell me things so I know you are interested in me.

- It's easier if you don't look at me too much – looking at a book or at my work makes me feel more comfortable.

- Let me know that if you ask questions it's OK for me to nod or shake my head at the moment.

- In News or Show-and-Tell time, I can show a photo or a drawing of things I've done at the weekend or in the holidays; or I can bring something in from home.

- Let me know that you won't ask me questions in front of the class unless I put my hand up."

COMMUNICATING MORE

"I'm starting to communicate in different ways, without speaking. It's not that I will always need to use signs or talking cards – I know that real talking is quicker and more fun – but at the moment:

- I need to get confident communicating silently by smiling, nodding and pointing before using my voice. I'm starting to use my fingers for numbers when we do sums too.

- I'm stuck when I need to say or ask something – like asking for help or to go to the toilet. Maybe I could have a sign or a picture I could use instead.

- Emotion symbols are useful to show you if I feel ill or someone has upset me.

- Now that I can write a bit more, could I use a dry-wipe board perhaps?

- I like it if we have to speak or answer all together – I say the words inside my head or even move my lips sometimes.

- Maybe my voice will come out if my face is hidden behind a mask or I can be the voice for a puppet."

TALKING ABOUT MY SM

"Of course, I'd like everyone to think I'm the same as other children – that I don't have this difficulty talking. But I guess they know I don't speak. So it's best if there's some talk about my SM.

- It helps if I know that all the teaching staff know that I've got SM – and that they understand about it and will treat me in the same way. Please ask them to tell me (quietly in private) that they know I find it hard sometimes to speak out. And that I can speak when I'm ready.

- I feel very stressed when there are supply teachers. Could you write something about me having SM to give them to read before they take our class?

- And could you tell the dinner ladies and playground people about SM? I don't think they have seen someone with it or understand about it.

- The other children make comments and ask questions about my SM. Please tell them a bit about SM – I'm sure my mum can help you with what to say if you want. Don't let them say I can't speak – I CAN speak, and WILL speak if everyone's patient."

REDUCING STRESS

"There are some things I find very stressful. But there are ways to help me.

- I could join in small group or class activities more easily if I knew at the start that no talking was needed.

- It's hardest for me to relax and talk when there are lots of people around. Could I have some special time with you or another teacher in the corner of the class or in another room – or maybe after school?

- It's awful when teachers tell me they wish I'd talk to them – so do I, but I can't at the moment. Some have even offered me a big reward when I speak, which, of course, I'd like but it feels totally out of reach.

- I'm not good with unexpected things because I'm afraid that I will be expected to talk more than I can. Please give me advance notice about changes, or things that don't usually happen – like a change in the timetable, or a different teacher.

- And I get in a special panic when I know I have to move to a new class with a new teacher. It'd be great if I could have extra preparation for this.

- I worry a lot about tests! If there are some coming up, please talk to me and my mum about the best way of tackling them."

HELPING ME WITH FRIENDS

"It's hard to make friends if you don't talk. I'm sure it seems rude or unfriendly – or perhaps it seems weird. Here are some ideas of how you might help me with my friends.

- To help me join in more, can you ask children to invite me to sit with them?

- Small groups are easier for me and some children seem to understand me better than others.

- It especially helps if my best friend, who I am talking to at my home, can be in the group.

- I get more worried if Maya is not in school. Can I sit with one of my 'next best friends' instead please?

- Please can you ask the other children to include me at playtime – just one or two to begin with until I can manage in a bigger group?

- It's awful when children push me to speak, or talk about me being silent. Can you help them to understand about SM, and not to talk about it?

- The worst thing is when they laugh at me or try and copy me. Please stop them doing this.

- I'm worried that when I start speaking they'll laugh or make a big deal of it. I'd like them to act normal and take no special notice."

SPECIFIC ACTIVITIES

Register

"I find it hard to answer the register. I get more and more panicky the closer it gets to my name. Perhaps we could give our answers in a different way – we could all nod or put our hand up when you say our name, or we could all answer together when you say each name."

Reading

"I can point if you want me to find words that you read out. Or I could match words to the right picture. And if we have to read in pairs, I can sometimes mouth the words or shake my head when my partner gets it wrong. If you want me to, I could read at home and my mum could tell you how I do – or perhaps she could record it."

Jobs

"I really like to join in things where I don't have to talk. Please give me a job – I could help decorate the classroom, tidy the books or hand out the pencils. Maybe I could help someone who's new or doesn't know how to do her job very well? I might even be able to take the register to the office if someone came with me at first."

Projects

"I could make a Talking Card or Book at home if we can agree on who can listen to the recording."

FEELING GOOD ABOUT MYSELF

"I often feel cross and upset at school because I can't talk freely. And I wish I could answer questions and tell you things so you know I am clever. I can't feel good about talking yet. Can you please help me feel good in other ways?

- It's great when you smile at me. I'm always looking out for it.

- I'd like to get more stickers for non-talking things I do. But please don't stick one on my jumper in case someone asks me what it's for.

- I feel proud when you tell people about good work I've done, but please don't draw attention to my talking targets.

- I really like art and music – I almost feel I can communicate through them. I'd like to be able to do more art and music with others who like it too."

HOME/SCHOOL LINKS

"With me having SM, I suppose we need the school to be extra helpful in some ways.

- Could we have a home–school message book to fill in the gap of me not talking yet?

- It might help if you came to my home and could see my room and the things I like and do there. We could play my favourite game.

- I'd like to think you and my mum and dad are friends and can talk about how best to help me with my SM.

- Maybe if I could come into school, or even into the playground, when the children are not there, that would help me feel less anxious at the beginning of the day.

- Could I come in early or stay behind on some days to talk to my mum and my little brother in the classroom, the library or another room?

- And could my mum or dad sometimes come into the classroom when the other children are there, or go on school trips with us? As I get used to talking to my parents in these places, other people can gradually get closer and join in."

SPECIAL DIFFICULTIES

Going to the toilet

"I used to try and hang on till I got home as I hated using the school toilet so much. Mum said that was why I got an infection and had to take medicine. Once I wet myself in the classroom, which was really embarrassing. But I'm managing better now.

- We agreed a system to show when I need to go to the toilet and you let me choose to use a picture or symbol, or make a signal.

- It helps if I go with Maya or another friend.

- And it's good if we can go first or when other kids are not there.

Mum found out that some children with SM are so anxious that they never use the school toilets. She said they need to have a special programme to help them get over it, starting with whatever they can manage, and gradually changing only one thing at a time."

Eating in school

"When I first came to school, I didn't feel very comfortable at lunchtime. It was something about being in the big hall and feeling that lots of people were watching me. My teacher let me eat my lunch with a small group of children in the classroom, and then we had our own table in the hall.

Some children have a big problem with this – a sort of eating phobia. They need a special small-steps programme for this too."

How parents can help

IMPORTANT THINGS TO REMEMBER

"Can I first tell you a few main things that I think might help us get over my SM quicker? They might not all be easy but it's good to have a chance to tell you:

- When you are relaxed about me and my speaking difficulty, it helps me feel more relaxed and happy too. And when I see you are stressed about it, my worries get worse.

- It panics me when you don't seem to know what to do. I need you to tell me it's not unusual to find talking difficult at times and reassure me that I will get better at it – just like you used to reassure me when I was afraid of the dark or couldn't ride my bike.

- Lots of people don't know about SM and say unhelpful things. When they are making it hard for me – putting on pressure to get me to talk, or making comments – please tell them what is going on and how to help me. Maybe they would like to read this book!

- I feel good when I hear you tell other people about things I'm good at – and I don't mind showing them things I find easy to do."

HELPING ME WITH MY WORRIES

"Sometimes I try not to talk about what bothers me because I think it will make you more worried.

And sometimes I get sad or very cross without really knowing why. It helps if you can:

- Let me talk a bit about my worries – not so I can get lots of sympathy (somehow that makes my worries seem even bigger), but so we can talk about what will help.

- Help me to work out a plan to manage, or to think of something that will be a comfort.

- Let me know what we are doing each day, especially if there are new or different things. When you don't warn me about surprises, I find myself worrying the whole time about what might happen next.

- Maybe act out things with me that we are going to do, like going to the doctor, or ordering food at the café.

- If lots and lots of worries are going round and round in my head, help me to draw or write them down; then we can decide if we need to focus on any of them today and how we are going to manage them.

- Give me some time when I get home to relax and chill after a stressful day at school. Sometimes going on the swing or the trampoline helps."

MOVING ME FORWARD

"It's not good for me to do nothing and avoid every sort of talking situation – I'll never improve, and the more I avoid things, the more scary they will seem. Please try and find a small way that I can join in.

- Perhaps I could go to a party for a short time at the beginning, rather than arrive and have to go into a room full of people or not go at all.

- In a restaurant maybe I could *show* the waiter what I want rather then tell him.

- I could say my Brownie promise at the same time as Maya – that way it won't matter if my voice is very quiet or only my lips are moving.

- I could write 'thank you' on paper shapes to give to friends and relatives.

- I could record a special message for Granddad's birthday as long as you promise you won't play it to anyone else without asking me first.

- Maybe I could record our answerphone message.

- My auntie could listen over the phone while I read to you.

- I could use our web-cam to have fun with my cousins, starting with games that don't need talking."

HELPING ME WITH MY FRIENDS

"I can't really relax with friends at school yet and I need some help to practise doing things with them outside school.

- As well as Maya, can I have one or two other friends round to our home?

- When they come, please don't just leave us all the time. It's best if we do some things with you for part of the time, especially at the beginning.

- I think it'd be good if we do things we like – cooking or something arty – where we don't have to talk but we can.

- Or maybe we can play outside or in the park; we could play on the swings, or go swimming.

- I don't want them to stay too long at first. So can you please agree a finish time with their mums?

- I notice other children enjoy messy play and don't mind getting their things in a muddle. I know it makes you anxious when I get dirty or make a mess, and this is making it hard for me to relax with other children. So can we please wait till the very end before we clean up?"

WITH WIDER FAMILY AND FRIENDS

"When we are with other people where I don't feel comfortable, there are things you do that can make it better or worse:

- Please give me some time to warm up with no one paying me attention or all looking at me.

- It helps if I can do something, join in or have a job that doesn't need talking.

- Please don't push me forward to speak or to perform.

- I feel very embarrassed if you comment on my talking difficulty when there's no need, but please warn people that I may be quiet but that's OK.

- I don't like you speaking for me as if I don't exist; or you saying something that's NOT what I want to say or do! It's not easy but it's better if I try to speak to you and then you can say it for me.

- Sometimes we need to move further away so I can talk to you face to face. Gradually we won't need to move so far away and I'll get used to talking to you properly in front of other people, rather than whispering in your ear

- I like it when we all say or sing things together – like 'Happy Birthday' – but don't look at me to see if I've joined in."

LINKS WITH SCHOOL AND OUTSIDE ACTIVITIES

"Here's how you can help me with things to do with school or outside-school activities:

- When you drop me off at school or ballet, don't make me promise to do some talking.

- And when you meet me afterwards, please don't ask me about what talking I've done, as though that's the most important thing and the only thing you are interested in.

- It's good when you come to help at school or at Brownies, especially when we go out on trips. But it works best when you help others too – not just stick with me.

- If I'm doing a new thing or going on a trip, that's a big step. I want to do it but am afraid I might not manage and may want to come back part way through. Could you make that all right with the teacher?

- I can't stick up for myself yet when kids are mean, so can we use a message book to let my teacher know if I'm having trouble?

THANK YOU for listening!"

Recommended reading, DVDs, resources, organisations and websites

BOOKS FOR PARENTS, TEACHERS AND OTHER ADULTS

Johnson, Maggie and Wintgens, Alison (2001) *The Selective Mutism Resource Manual.* Milton Keynes: Speechmark Publishing.

Shipon-Blum, Elisa (2003) *The Ideal Classroom Setting for the Selectively Mute Child.* Philadelphia: Dr E. Shipon-Blum and Selective Mutism Anxiety Research and Treatment Center.

McHolm, Angela E., Cunningham, Charles E. and Vanier, Melanie K. (2005) *Helping Your Child with Selective Mutism.* Oakland, CA: New Harbinger Publications.

BOOKS FOR CHILDREN AND YOUNG PEOPLE

Longo, Sharon L. (2006) *My Friend Daniel Doesn't Talk.* Milton Keynes: Speechmark Publishing.
Targeted at 4–8-year-olds, this book will help teachers explain Selective Mutism to the whole class.

Dunbar, Polly (2007) *Penguin.* London: Walker Books.
Young children and adults alike will laugh out loud at this book, which beautifully illustrates what will not help children to speak!

Kent, Trilby (2009) *Medina Hill.* Toronto, ON: Tundra Books.
Eleven-year-old Dominic has SM and is the hero of this adventure, which is set in 1935.

Thorpe, Jessica (2011) *Slipping in and out of my Two Worlds.* Lulu online publishing: www.lulu.com
Beautifully written by a 19-year-old who has overcome the condition, this uplifting coming-of-age story pulls no punches in highlighting the agonies of living with SM in teenage years.

DVD

Silent Children: Approaches to Selective Mutism (2004). Available from SMIRA (see below). Produced jointly with Leicester University School of Education.
This excellent 24-minute film includes moving testimonials from recovered survivors of SM, and will help adults and children alike to understand and manage the condition.

RESOURCES
Talking Products
www.talkingproducts.co.uk
Phone: 02380 730 731

ORGANISATIONS AND WEBSITES
UK
The Selective Mutism Information and Research Association (SMIRA)
c/o 5 Keyham Close,
Leicester
LE5 1FW
www.smira.org.uk
Email: info@selectivemutism.co.uk
Phone: 08002289765

USA
The Selective Mutism Foundation
www.selectivemutismfoundation.org

Selective Mutism Group – Child Anxiety Network
www.selectivemutism.org

Canada
The Selective Mutism Network
www.selectivemutismnetwork.org

New Zealand
Selective Mutism Parent Support Group
Email: sm.info@nzord.org.nz

France
Ouvrir la Voix
www.ouvrirlavoix.sitego.fr

Italy

Associazione Italiana Mutismo Selettivo (AIMuSe)

www.aimuse.it

Norway

Mutisme.no – Foreningen selektiv mutisme

www.selektivmutisme.no

Sweden

Föreningen selektiv mutism

www.selektivmutism.se

Denmark

Selektiv mutisme

www.selektiv-mutisme.dk

Germany

Mutismus Selbsthilfe Deutschland e.V

www.mutismus-selbsthilfe.de

Switzerland

Mutismus Schweiz

www.mutismus.ch/de

Worldwide

Selective Mutism EU

www.selective-mutism.eu